B"h

Moshe Bernstein

Internet addiction

The complete guide to overcome the most
common addiction

Moshe Bernstein   2014

I.s.b.n -978-965-92222-0-9

1

Introduction

The internet age brought huge breakout in many fields. Scientists, students and research are using this tool. Day by day it is becoming an inseparable part of our life. There are many positive aspects of this media and much benefit can be gained from it. But there is also another side to this enormous wealth that the internet brought with it.

Many studies show that people's enslavement to the net is growing steadily. Taking part in Social networks, online games and the profusion of news and stimuli offered by the net increases every day. Accordingly there is an increase on the time that people spend on them.

Other studies reports uncontrolled use of the internet. The inability to pull away from surfing the net, the obsession that accompanies the use, and the multifaceted damage that it causes bear witness that these are forms of addiction.

Recently, a new definition has been added to the field: I.A.D. Internet Addiction Disorder. According to experts in the field, this addiction could become one of the most common disorders.

Some people argue that internet addiction controls them and they are unable to get away from it. It is tempting to think this way, but the reality is completely different. Our control over our lives is in our hands alone. The key for change depends on our way of perception and emotion. We are the ones who control how we think and the way we feel. We can definitely have the choice to control our habits when surfing the internet.

If we change our thinking and emotional patterns, we will make a significant change in the way we relate to life events, our moods, personal communication, and other aspects of our lives. The guiding principle is that the choice is in our hands. These goals of developing awareness, and correctly managing the way we think and feel stand at the base of the process of achieving control over our habits when using the internet.

Addiction is often linked to a chemical imbalance in the brain. Recent research shows significant similarities in the characteristics of the chemical reactions in the brains of drug-addicts and alcoholics and those of people suffering internet addiction! The neurological mechanism of addiction is similar in almost all addictions. This is the case either in the use of psycho-active substances or in the case of behavioral addiction like the internet addiction.

It is important to emphasize that the processes described in the book are not only meant for those addicted to the internet. Almost anyone can achieve a significant improvement, a higher sense of self-control and an inner feeling of wholeness.

Self-help books have gained momentum in past years and become more and more popular. This is a self-help book, although in extreme cases, or if there is a disorder, there is no substitute for traditional treatment either face to face or in support groups that works the 12 steps program. If it is known that there are additional problems like depression or anxiety, it is advisable to contact a professional therapist.

Moshe Bernstein

Contents

Basic Concepts

Internet addiction and uncontrolled surfing is one of the most common problems these days. In many countries the scale of internet dependence and obsessive surfing habits is growing even among children. This sounds rather frightening, but before you get despair and run off to surf the net, please listen! Internet addiction is a problem that can be challenged. It will not always be a part of you. The problem is not the person; the problem is the real problem! The methods in this book give a way to find real improvement and to give you better control over your life. In support groups for addiction it is usually said that you are not responsible for getting into the problem, but it *is* your responsibility to get *out* of it.

Is it the internet itself that is the problem? The internet itself is a wonderful tool for important, beneficial uses, and it can be wonderful if it used properly. The problem comes up with the way it is used. When obsessive use of the net comes at the expense of important things like work, family relationships, study, or sport, then it is clear that there is a problem with surfing habits and this could point to addictive behavior. Some say that addictive characteristics are only possible with substance abuse like that of alcohol and drugs, but there has been a few studies on behavioral addictions that take place without psycho-active substances, like addiction to computer games, gambling addiction and compulsive overeating.

What is addiction? Addiction is defined as the development of dependence on an addictive substance, or actions and behaviors that are done over and over again for thrills. There are some studies that show that tendency of some people to develop dependency or even addiction to chemical substances comes from interpersonal crises that are either family or work related. Others claim that a genetic structure is related to this tendency. It is quite common to find additional cases of addiction in the same family.

In the short term, addiction improves the mood and general feeling of a person. It reduces anxiety and raises self esteem and gives a feeling of wholeness. In the long term, addiction damages quality of life, demands increasing resources and causes a physical, mental and financial draining out. Addiction demands that a person spend more and more time on it. The priorities of an addict change. The addiction becomes the centre of his life. It becomes his first and foremost priority, and harms important parts of life like family, social life, work or studies. While he is busy surfing the net, the addict experiences reduction in the negative feelings that bother him, but after a while he feels feelings of guilt, shame and frustration. This becomes a vicious cycle that influences and enslaves his whole life. The addict is in an unstoppable obsession. He has to be constantly online and always connected. If there is suddenly a communication problem he feels that it's the end of the world. The lack of inner serenity, the constant rush after new thrills and the ongoing flow of constantly surfing the net becomes part of his life even when he is not sitting in front of the computer. he waits impatiently for the moment when he can again sit in front of the screen. The addict is in a state of constant dissatisfaction. This feeling causes him feelings of frustration and a wish to find compensation that will ease his negative feelings. It is like a barrel that we are trying to fill with water. The problem is that there is a hole in the bottom of the barrel. All our attempts to fill the barrel will fail. We will always have to fill it more and more. Some of them feel that they are like a bottomless pit. There is never a real feeling of satisfaction or tranquility. There is always an urge to find a new excitement. This constant dissatisfaction and rush for excitement can lead us to places we did not expect.

There are a few levels of internet addiction.

On a Physical level there is a compulsive, strong urge to surf the internet. Usually an addict will find sophisticated ways to justify himself. This can come at the expense of others. The life of the addict becomes out of control and ruled by his addiction.

On a mental level the brain of the addict is full of obsessive thoughts and longings for continued addictive internet use. The addiction becomes part of his life and without it, his life seems empty and meaningless. A double life, denial, self-delusion and lies are part of the behavior of an addict. His emotional world shrinks and it becomes difficult for him to express his feelings. There is a reduction in personal functions, and the way he relates to his surroundings.

On a spiritual level the addict is focused only on his own needs. Sometimes he will be very selfish with others. All his mental energy is dedicated to his addiction and almost no energy left for positive action in other areas of life. The addict has no spiritual content in his life and does not feel he is connected to a Higher Power.

In some ways Internet Addiction is more problematic than addiction to drugs or alcohol. The availability and accessibility of the internet is part of the problem. It is much easier to gain access to the internet in compare to alcohol and drugs. Internet usage is legal, where alcoholism or any use of drugs is a crime. Drugs and alcohol are greatly more expensive than an internet connection. Alcohol and drugs use considered a problem of people who are low on the socio-economic scale. Internet addiction is not stigmatized or associated with any class of people. Here we find the real danger. In an innocent disguise, the internet sneaks into our lives without being aware of the deft of the problem that can influence and affect our whole life.

In the general definition of internet addiction, there are a few sub-groups:

Gambling- Gambling with sums of money in an on-line casino. This also includes speculative dealings in shares and foreign currency by people who are not trained for this. The statistics shows that beginners lose all their money on the stock market.

Games- Addiction to on-line gaming on the internet.

Social Networks- This group is obsessively busy with social interactions on the net, connecting with other people and making new internet friends.

Cybersex Addiction– compulsive use of Internet pornography, adult chat rooms, fantasy role-play sites, chat rooms, and messaging that impact negatively on real-life relationships with your family and friends. The result is that virtual online friends, become more important than your family and friends in the real world.

News- An endless race to be constantly updated by news on news-sites on a range of topics financial news, sports and others.

Looking for thrills is usually an outcome of boredom and a feeling of emptiness. Sometimes the endless run for satisfaction and excitement can be linked to an inner experience of deprivation, something that leads us in an endless search, where we are trying to balance this inner lack with excitement. Here we see the paradox where this constant running after satisfaction and excitement only strengthens and amplifies the negative feelings.

The processes described in the book are likely to bring you to a number of goals:

Better control over your internet surfing habits and real relief from symptoms of compulsive internet usage.

Awareness and understanding about what happens inside yourself. You will know what things you need to avoid. This awareness of what happens inside your heart and soul and the processes that are happening within you will allow you to make good use of your inner energies in more useful areas.

Taking responsibility for oneself-You are the only one responsible for what is happening with you. Instead of trying to solve the problem in a way that will only sink you deeper into obsession and addiction you will learn to take responsibility upon yourself, using the power of self-choice. In this way you will be able to control and manage yourself in an effective way and not be managed by unwanted forces.

Preservation - Real abstinence in the long term.

Are my internet surfing habits normal?

Man has always been curious, with ambition to learn more and more. In childhood, children's learn many things as a result of their natural curiosity. This curiosity is an important attribute for learning and progress. From this perspective, the internet has wide almost unlimited possibilities to satisfy human curiosity and learning. There is almost no field that one cannot find information on the internet. Many scientific research projects were done with the aid of the internet and the net's contribution to science and research is tremendous. But what is the difference between useful surfing and obsessive out of control surfing.

There are a few crucial differences.

The need Is it really necessary to surf the internet now? Is it serving a positive purpose like study, education or recreation? Will it serve one of my areas of life in a constructive fashion?

Harm to family and relationships. Is the amount of time that we devote to the internet harm our family closeness? Are we ignoring family members? Are we hearing complaints from them about the amount of time we are spending on the net? Is this causing a rift in the family? Will this internet use cause arguments and fights within the family? Are the children being neglected?

Has this internet usage become something that rules us? In a state of addiction the addict loses control of himself and his life becomes ruled by his addiction. Is this true in our case? Has this surfing gotten out of hand and out of our control?

Have there been numerous attempts to stop and then again you have fallen into the same pattern? Do you have feelings of remorse and shame after using the net? Do we lose the feeling of time passing when we are surfing the internet? Does it happen that we look at the watch and suddenly realize that "its already four in the morning and I didn't feel the hours go by"?

Are other areas of our life being damaged? Is this obsessive internet surfing coming at the expense of other parts of life? Are our studies and other tasks being neglected as a result of our habits? Is our work suffering? Is our boss no longer satisfied with us because we are exhausted after long nights of spending time on the internet? Do you push off tasks and assignments only because you are busy on the internet?

These criteria are in effect the major differences between internet use that is constructive and useful, that benefits our life, empowering us, and letting us progress; and the compulsive addictive form of use that rules us and in effect paralyzes our everyday function in all aspects of our life.

Addiction to internet surfing on Smartphones

Smartphones are intruding into more and more Aspects of our life and for some of us they have long ago become some sort of sly drug. The enormous amount of information that flows from the various applications can bring us a lot of benefit. But sometimes, there is an addictive influence. How many times a day do you take up the phone and you find yourself looking at the screen? Are the amount of time you look at the screen increasing? Do you find yourself even in the middle of driving automatically taking out the phone and looking at what's happening there? Does it happen that in the middle of a meal or a meeting you find yourself checking what is happening on the social networks? How many times in the middle of lesson, when the lecturer becomes boring we take out our phones and write messages? Sometimes because of boredom or disinterest our instinctive reaction is to take out our cell phone? For many people it has already become an automatic, unconscious way of acting. A sort of bad habit that its hard to get rid of. Many of us have tried to get ride off this complete dependency on our smartphones but find out very soon that the addiction is much stronger than we are. The social networks have become dominant in the life of many people and there are many who feel alone when they are off. The dependency is so strong that being cut off from their social network or from the internet in general, they experience a feeling of nervousness, discomfort and anxiety. Linking up to their social networks will relieve their feelings of loneliness and the unconscious fear of being "alone". This fear of loneliness is sometimes so strong that the need for social interaction on the internet becomes actually addictive over time and being linked constantly to friends that gives a feeling of security and social acceptance. As long as this social experience does not adversely influence real life, there is no problem, because at the end of the day, social acceptance is one of our needs as human beings. But what happens if we are abandoning part of our duties in favor of this virtual social experience? Perhaps there is overdependence on this social endorsement? Am I constantly in need of this endorsement by my virtual friends to feel that I exist, I am a success, clever, funny and others? What happens when central functions of my life like work, quality time with the family, regular exercise, are damaged by this addiction to it? When other areas of life are being harmed, we have to ask ourselves if we haven't crossed the red line between beneficial activities with friends and our social life.

How to diagnose internet addiction.

Are you addicted to the internet? Is there a real problem or is this in fact normative behavior? It is very important that you know your exact situation in the most accurate way. The term "addict" is one we associate with a wretched man you might find on the streets. "It's for sure not me." Many think. This is where the problem lies.

Addiction can happen to anyone. It can also happen to those who seem to be successful, intelligent and talented.

Take a few minutes to fill in this questionnaire. When you are done, you will get an assessment of whether or not you are addicted to the internet and what is the degree of the problem. In addition, after getting the results, you will know by the degree of the problem if you can be helped by this book in order to treat the problem, or it would be wise to get help from a professional therapist.

Questionnaire for assessing Internet Addiction

Near each question, write the score using the following key

0- never

1- almost never

2- seldom

3- sometimes

4- often

5- always

	0	1	2	3	4	5
Do you stay on the internet for longer than you planned?						
How many times did it happen that you signed on with virtual ID and not with your own						

name?						
Does it happen that you prefer to surf the internet instead of enjoying yourself with your family?						
Do you make contact with other people on the net?						
Does your family complain about the amount of time you spend on the internet?						
Are your marks or your or work performance deteriorating as a result of the time you spend on the internet?						
Do you very frequently check your email?						
Do you wait for the						

moment when you can go online again?					
Do you form intimate relationships on the internet?					
Are you afraid that your life without internet will be boring?					
Do you become angry when someone disturbs you while you are online?					
Are you losing sleep because you are using the internet at all hours?					
Do you find yourself saying to others: "in a minute" when you are using the internet?					
Have you tried, and failed to cut down on the					

time you spend on internet use?						
Do you choose to go online instead of enjoying yourself with friends?						
Do you feel that you are missing something when you are not online?						
Does your negative feelings relieve when you sit down to surf the net?						

Total points:

20 points or less: The internet really doesn't interest you. You're fine.

40-20 points: You are still okay. You don't usually go overboard.

60-40 points: The internet interrupts your life.

60 points and over: It is likely that here there is an addiction to the internet.

75 points and over: Do you ever leave the computer?!

If you got over 60 points in this test then you need to do something beyond your own efforts that you put into finding a solution to this problem. You need to get help and professional assistance. This can be support groups, a psychologist who is expert in the field of addiction, or a social worker who specialized in treating addiction. Don't stay alone with this problem. The price that you pay for it is too high.

Characteristics of Internet Addiction

The most prominent characteristics of internet addiction:

1. Repeated attempts to get out from this overdependence on the internet that usually end in failure. This causes a feeling of distress.

2. The dependency increases over time. The need for a level of excitement. There is an irresistible urge to carry on.

3. A loss of the sense of time passing when using the internet. Staying at the computer deep into the night.

4. Neglect of commitments to work, studies and business.

5. Neglect of commitments to family and spouse.

6. In spite of the damage done by the addiction the addict continues to surf the internet and makes no change in his habits.

7. Time is spent thinking about and planning internet use when one is not online.

8. In the case where there is no opportunity to surf the net, the addict develops a feeling of longing and yearning for being online again.

9. Damage to daily functions because of the addiction.

10. There is a denial that there is any problem. The addict refuses to acknowledge that he has a

problem and so anyway refuses or is too scared to help himself.

Using the internet does in fact sometimes provide excitement and the feelings of shelter from reality. But when we escape into a virtual landscape, a new problem comes up. this problem can burden a person's life and disrupt it. Important daily tasks can be pushed aside as a result of all the time spent in front of the computer screen. Addictive use of the internet is usually related to denial on the part of the addict. Have you ever tried to speak to an internet addict when he is online? Any attempt to talk to him will cause an angry reaction like: "Leave me alone " or "Don't disturb me right now". Internet addiction has an overwhelmingly negative effect on a couple's relationship. The marital loyalty of a couple may be harmed as a result of one of the spouses making use of social networks or dating sites. The ability to have relationships directly over the internet is a formidable threat to the stability of the couple as a unit. More and more mental energies and reserves are turned towards virtual interactions instead of time being spent with the family. As a result of this, important family relationships in the addicted person's life are damaged because of the ongoing surfing. The net cause's chronic tiredness, a decline in memory, lowered levels of production and general functioning and causes frustration and disappointment and maybe even "jealousy" because the addicted person is ignoring those surrounding him. Functioning at work can also suffer and many addicted people are fired from their jobs.

Has it happened to you that you find you have lost track of time and suddenly you see that it is three or four in the morning, and you have to get up at six to start a new day? You will definitely not be wide awake the next day. Losing sense of time is very much a characteristic of addictive situations. The addict "finds" himself still online without meaning to be so at four and five in the morning and even then he finds it difficult to drag himself away. Even when he gets up to do other things, his brain is still burning with thoughts about how and when he will be able to reconnect to the internet and continue his addictive surfing.

A distinguishing quality of addiction is dependency. The addicted person becomes progressively dependent on his link to the internet. He finds that he cannot control himself and is not able to even think about disconnecting himself from the internet. He sees his internet usage as being integral with his personality. He has the notion that separating him from the internet would be like amputating a finger. These negative beliefs that are found often in the minds of addicted people become self-fulfilling prophesy.

The motivation to carry out everyday tasks weakens and the only drive that remains to the person is to continue surfing the internet. His lifestyle focuses on and revolves around his internet connection and leaves no available energy for meaningful emotional investments in his family and in other areas of life. The addicted person lives in a sort of survival even in his day to day life only to keep his alternate world. A virtual universe that he has built within his addiction.

Use of the internet for actual positive, legitimate purposes is not the problem at all. The internet can serve a useful, beneficial purpose. The problem with uncontrolled use that it interferes with a person's function on the daily life. Procrastination putting off tasks becomes worse and many important tasks are not done because most of the time is spent in front of the screen.

The urge or the craving to continue surfing obsessively has been described many times as tough and impossible to control. As is the case with all addictions, the main difficulty is how to deal with the intense craving that can suddenly come upon the person. Later on we will discuss ways to deal with these urges and cravings. One efficient way to deal with it is to call a friend or someone who is part of your support system and talk to him about your difficulty. Another way to manage it is to give yourself over to a Higher Power. The addicted person admits to his own helplessness in the face of his addiction and gives himself over to a beneficent Higher Power who can help him.

Does it happen that you neglect and push off important matters in your life in order to surf the internet? Does it happen that your personal relationships with important figures in your life, in your family circle, or your work colleagues is disrupted?

34

Are the people close to you angry and very frustrated as a result of the many hours that you stay on the computer?

Does it happen that you react scary and defensively when people comment on your internet habits?

Do you have feelings of guilt and anxiety about your internet habits?

Does the internet serve as a way to keep you away from contact with people you don't like to be with or to remove off unpleasant feelings?

Has it happened when you tried to stop your obsessive surfing that you felt emptiness or emotional distress?

If the answer to most of these questions is "yes" then you have to get treatment.

Denial

Have you ever asked an addicted person if he admits to the fact that he is addicted?

Almost certainly the answer would be something like: "Nonsense! If I wanted to, I could get out of this easily." Or, "What's the problem here? Surfing the internet is not a problem at all!" or perhaps, "Oh, please! Why are you making an issue out of this? I could stop in one minute!"

This denial is a prominent characteristic of an addicted person. He uses psychological defense mechanisms to bear the fact that he is addicted, and also to keep on with his addiction in spite of the huge price he pay for it. This denial hides the bitter truth from the addict: You have lost control of your life! You are controlled and directed by compulsive behavior!

For an addicted person, this situation seems not real. He will make every effort to prove that this is not the case, he is convinced that he is in fact in control. He will justify himself.

Time after time you can hear addicted people who announce that if they just wanted they could stop at the same day.

Denial prevents the addicted person from facing the fact that he has been trapped by his internet habits. This denial allows him to continue his way of life despite the damage that caused by his addiction. It leaves the addicted person unaware of the severity of his problem.

It might be that he doesn't want to be aware of it. The addicted person ignores the ever increasing warning signs.

These warning signs can take the shape of fights with parents, arguments with a partner, an angry boss, neglected health issues or tests failed because of obsessive internet use.

Larry was a contractor who one night discovered the online games. They captured his heart. He especially loved the high-tension, exciting games. These games helped him to forget his usual grey day to day existence. With time, Larry felt he was being drawn into these games. He spent more and more hours on them but he convinced himself that this was "nothing".

Larry's wife began to say that she was uncomfortable with the way things were going but it did not help very much.

Larry maintained that these were just innocent games and he did not see them as a problem. In time, Larry's income suffered, because of all the time he was devoting to gaming. His marriage deteriorated to the point of divorce. At this point his wife's family got involved and demanded that he go and get professional treatment. Larry continued to deny that he need such treatment. Only when his wife actually sued for divorce Larry went to a therapist but continue to claim that he did not have any problem. Larry gradually begins to understand the depth of his denial.

Larry's behavior is typical for many addicts. Denial of the problem is a significant stumbling block in the way of rehabilitation. The mechanisms of denial do not allow the person to see that he has a problem. As the situation of an addicted person becomes progressively worse, he still refuses to admit that he have a problem and to begin any kind of treatment.

These are some of the characteristics of internet addiction. The purpose of this book is to give you tools to improve your control over your internet surfing habits so that you can manage your life better.

What does it give us?

What are people looking for on the internet? What does it give them? What is so powerful about the internet that draws so many people of all ages to it like a magnet?

An enormous data base.

The access to an infinite information excites the imagination. Almost anything can be found here. From recipes to scientific research. Our inborn human curiosity can find expression in boundless information in many fields of knowledge.

Virtual personality

We are not always what we want to be in our life many of us have unfulfilled dreams. These can be childhood ambitions, dream for wealth, and other wishes that are buried deep inside us. On the internet we can remove the shackles and limitations of our real selves. Here we are given the opportunity to build a new personality.

Easing the pain

Many people suffer emotional pain. There can be reasons for that. This pain is not expressed in daily life but it stays there deep inside and sometimes bubbles up. In this instance, surfing the internet can act as a pain reliever.

Low self esteem

For people who have low self-esteem, the internet with its forums and social groups can act as a compensation for their low self-esteem. Here they are free of the bindings of embarrassment and poor self confidence and they can feel more accepted and equal to others.

Loneliness

It is not secret that in Western Society there is a high percentage of lonely people. In this case the internet sometimes serves as a tool against loneliness, and to give a sense of social connection. Joining forums and social groups on the internet keep away loneliness. A feeling of loneliness does not strictly affect people living alone. Many people who are part of a family unit or a social circle can still feel alone even in a group. Finding a sense of belonging on the internet can fulfill the needs of these people.

Gratification and excitement
On the internet one can find a wide spectrum of sites that can satisfy ones search for all kinds of gratification and excitement. Everything is immediately and easily available and usually free.

Coping with boredom
For many people, boredom is a problem. The internet is a marvelous solution for them. One can find an endless supply of interesting topics. An excellent way to challenge boredom.

The Seeds of Disaster

The awareness to the factors that can cause addiction is very important. In this case they can be compared to rays of sunlight that just by the fact that they shed light it allows the plants to grow and develop. Release from the addiction and personal growth is both bound together. Developing a high level of self awareness is necessary

Almost every instance of addiction begins with the attempt to solve some personal problem. Encountering unpleasant situations in life can be a motivating force behind an action that will cause one to run away from the stress. The result only worsens it.

Rudy was a simple worker. He did not enjoy his job and dreamed of getting rich quickly. One day he found an internet gambling site that he liked. He began gambling with small amounts but gradually began to increase the sums. He felt excitement that he could win large sums of money in short time. Very soon he had lost all the money.

Rudy now felt that he must somehow get his money back and then stop gambling. He began borrowing money in order to continue gambling. Thus he found himself in a vicious, cruel and negative cycle of disappointment with his loses and then again gambling hoping to regain some of his original losses. Only after he had lost a lot of money over a long time his family revealed his gambling. It caused a very serious crisis that caused Rudy to go in for rehabilitation in a 12 step program. Then, He stopped gambling on the internet and with time returned to a normative lifestyle.

What are the main factors that would cause a person to become addicted to the internet? Have you ever asked yourself what forces push us down the slope into addiction?

Negative Feelings

Anxiety, depression and low self esteem can bring a person to escape to a place that will allow him to compensate. Pressure, tension, sadness, moods, low satisfaction and frustration are unpleasant emotions. Surfing the internet can be used as a compensation mechanism that covers over these types of negative feelings.

A lot of people live with feelings of loneliness. Participating in internet social groups can blunt this loneliness in the short term, but in the long term strengthens it because the person becomes isolated from the real world. In order to heal these feelings the internet forms a sort of screen that hides these feelings from us. It is very important to correctly diagnose these cases; are there other emotional problems in the background of this addictive internet surfing?

Negative life experiences

Everyone experiences something in their lives that leaves behind an imprint of pain. Addicts have a large amount of inner pain. The pain that comes from negative life experiences grows and strengthens through the years to something more than the original experience itself. The unconscious way to deal with this pain is to sometimes escape to a different world, an alternative reality that lets them forget this pain. This alternative world is much less demanding and hurtful than the real world. Unfortunately, this way will only intensify the pain, frustration and disappointment so that there is a vicious, negative cycle that intensifies the addiction.

Lack of social relations

Everyone wants good relations with other people. The human need to unite with something bigger than us that will give us confidence, wholeness and harmony. Those who do not have good social skills will turn the interaction on the internet to fill in what is missing in their daily life. In this case the internet serves as a social tool to compensate them for lack of social skills

happiness and joy

Experience of being part of and flowing with something large and infinite that accepts you as you are. Something that fills us in exciting content and lets us forgets the day to day life. The internet gives us this experience almost without limits. During the time of surfing the net, the person is unaware of himself, he is entirely connected to something outside of himself that encompasses him and lets him forget the world.

Craving for Excitement

The internet offers a large scale of opportunities for excitement. Dating sites and chat rooms, online game sites, gambling sites that provide online gambling opportunities and more. The common of all these is the high level of excitement that is provided. This type of surfing is characterized by an uncontrolled urge that is far beyond reasonable bounds that are recognized in the real world.

Boredom

Running away from a feeling of boredom or a feeling of frustration, can be standing at the basis of over using the internet in an uncontrolled manner. The attempt to run away from the unpleasant feelings can cause a loss of control over the internet use. It acts as a screen for a deeper problem.

An inexhaustible craving for new information in real time.

In this case one can take note of surfing news and gossip sites. Jumping from topic to topic and from site to site without any focus.

personal needs

Attention, appreciation, love, social interaction, acceptance, all these are examples of real needs. When the world does not supply these basic needs, or only gives them partially, a deficiency results. The automatic reaction can be escaping in to a virtual world. There this lack could be challenged. Some people have negative opinion on their physical image and this causes them low self esteem and difficulty in accepting themselves. In these cases, the addiction to the net and the virtual universe is a sort of defense mechanism that skip over the difficulties.

In order to be more efficient in our identification of the problem let us use the following model. First, we will identify our main needs. It could be that there are a few of them. After that we will try to understand which feelings or emotional distresses cause the problem. Then we will find the hot point which is the main pain point. Was it because of online gambling sites? Was it a family crisis that we experienced that sent us to a certain type of internet site? After that we need to find an inner willing to change our negative thought patterns that led us down in to addiction. The end result will be choosing more realistic, practical solutions in order to deal with what is lacking in us and be conscious of and aware of the fact that internet addiction is not a solution but a problem by itself.

Please read the following:

Identifying personal deficiencies

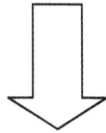

Identifying emotional distress and key beliefs that arise from it

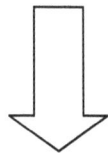

Have there been mistaken solutions?

↓

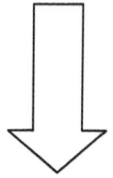

Describe them: Internet gambling, social networks, gaming, pornography etc.

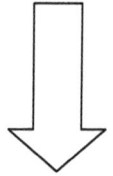

↓

A willingness to change old thought patterns and dealing with the deficiency

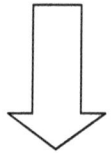

↓

Choosing a good solution, getting used to a new, constructive way of thinking

Usually there is a connection between the types of emotional problem to the type of internet addiction. For example, a poor worker who has many debts is likely to be drawn to gambling sites, and at the same time, a lonely person will be using the social networks. Everyone likes to feel that he is a winner. In real life we cannot always be winners. Gaming, besides the excitement it generates can also fulfill this need to be a winner in the virtual world. Marital problems and relationship difficulties can cause escape in to the virtual world in order to form new relationships. This acts as a compensation for the disappointments in the real life relationships. If couples are uncomfortable in their relationships, they may look for support, acceptance and comfort in chat rooms and social networks. There they will try to be in a comforting, non-threatening atmosphere. The fact that they do not have to expose their identities helps them to build up their imaginary characters. They will use it to fulfill their wishes they cannot achieve in the real world. With an imaginary identity, the addicted person can put aside many norms of real life. His hands are not tied by ethical standards and codes. The internet is a tool that allows access. This access sometimes encourages behavior that perhaps would never develop in the real world.

Rona experienced a bad childhood when she lost her mother at an early age. She also had a complicated relationship with her husband. One night she discovered the social networks and within a short time her entire life and schedule has been changed. She rotated around this new world she had discovered. A lot of Conversations in chat rooms and on her cell-phone. She sent and received tens and hundreds of messages a day. Her virtual friendships became more and more defendant and she began to meet some of them. She neglected her work and her children and spent most of her time on these relationships. One day, Rona's husband found out everything and it caused a huge crisis. Her job was in real danger. At this stage she went in to a rehabilitation program and went through a long, deeply personal process of self-discovery.

During this time, Rona detached herself from the social networks and started to help new addicted women at the start of their journey to recovery.

Internet addiction is a kind of safe heaven .it creates a vicious, negative cycle that feeds and intensifies itself as time goes by. Trying to soothe emotional distress by using compensating addictive behavior is like trying to fight fire with jet fuel. The person develops additional problems in his day to day functioning because of the addiction and so the need for a compensating mechanism arises again. The artificial solution to the problem only magnifies the addiction. This diagram will illustrate the cruel cycle that the internet addict gets caught up in. Internet surfing is a kind of "do it yourself" solution for distressing problems that in fact causes greater difficulties.

Ed was addicted to online gambling. In his heart he felt uncomfortable with his actions. He felt guilty about neglecting his work and family and about putting so much money into gambling. After a series of losses, he decided to stop all gambling! He thought the willpower is enough to stop and to overcome the urge to gamble. One night, after a loud argument with his wife, he went online and gambled with a small sum. Than he lose control. Another gamble and another until he found himself out of control. before dawn, when he remembered his decision not to gamble he got up and left the computer. Then, immediately began to think "I am a hopeless case" These thoughts led him to deep disappointment so that the only thing he could do to calm himself down was to go back to the gambling sites.

In the famous children's story, "The Little Prince" written by author Antoine Exupery, (1943), the little prince finds alcoholic and tries to help him:

> "Why are you drinking?" the
> little prince asked.
> "In order to forget" replied
> the drunkard.

"To forget what?" enquired the little prince, who was already feeling sorry for him.

"To forget that I am ashamed" the alcoholic confessed, hanging his head.

"Ashamed of what?" asked the little prince who wanted to help him.

"Ashamed of drinking!" concluded the drunkard, withdrawing into total silence.

And the little prince went away, puzzled.

"Grown-ups really are very, very odd", he said to himself as he continued his journey.

— Antoine Exupéry,
The Little Prince

The person addicted to the internet is trapped in a negative cycle. He does not want to be enslaved. Because of shame and disappointment he sinks deeper and deeper. This trap needs to be identified. One needs to be aware of the way it works and to learn how to overcome it.

By admitting his helplessness in the face of his addiction he has reached the first stage of his recovery.

An addicted person cannot overcome his problem just using his own willpower. He will need the help of something stronger than him and stronger than his addiction to jump out of the swamp.

Further on we will get to know the 12 steps recovery program.

Everything is in your Head

You are standing in line at the supermarket and suddenly someone tries to push and jump in front of you. A   loud argument breaks out. The other shoppers remain calm and quiet. Why does one person react in one way while others are staying calm? The main answer resides in the way we interpret events. We don't always have control over events that happen around us. We do, however, have control over the way we interpret them. The more realistic the interpretation is, the less we will be affected. If we take things personally, then we *will* be affected!

Many events happen over the course of our life. Some of these are key events, important parts of our life history. Others are only insignificant life situations. Our reactions to all these events will depend on the way we interpret them. This is why it is very important to practice how to interpret events in an objective manner. This will minimize the chance of distorted interpretations that lead to negative feelings that come with this kind of subjective commentary. Take note of the order of events:

An outside event that is not in our control, or another person's actions.

Thoughts- this is where our interpretation comes in to play and this *is* under our control! Either we can think thoughts like: "How he dare do that?",

"Why does he think that he's more important than anyone else?", *or* we can choose not to identify the event as a threat and then think to ourselves: "Is this really worth getting upset about?"

Feelings- After the thoughts negative feelings come Frustration, helplessness etc. If we have interpreted the event in an objective manner then our feelings will be more balanced.

Behavior- This can be shouting and anger, *or* if the interpretation was objective, the reaction will be calm and balanced. When we learn how to interpret events it will prevent the negative feelings. Knowing how to interpret things is necessary to achieve emotional balance. We do not want to spend our life in bitterness and energy. We dedicate all energies for good, constructive purposes.

Stress- Managing stress correctly begins with spotting the sources of stress in our lives. This is not always an easy task. The real roots of mental stress are not always clear to us and are sometimes under the surface, beneath the levels of consciousness. Sometimes we need to be made aware of these stressors.

Do you have frequent outbursts? Do you blame others or random events for the stress you are under?

An important aspect of the process is the recognition that taking personal responsibility for anger management is one of the most necessary steps for gaining control over our levels of stress.

There are many ways to mange stress. Some of these ways are helpful and constructive, and some are destructive. One of the ways to alleviate stress is by obsessive use of the internet. This is a compensatory mechanism that comes as a reaction to our emotional imbalance. This is why it is so important to learn how to manage our stress levels and to deal with them in a healthy manner. Recovery from internet addiction is related with problems that are under the surface. These can be problems like depression, anxiety, trauma, or perhaps an inability to manage emotions properly.

What can we do to prevent unnecessary stress?

A lot can be done.

First of all, we need to change our thoughts and emotional patterns.

Keep away from people and situations that cause stress- If you know that there are certain people who cause you stress, keep away from them as much as possible. If getting involved in hot political arguments raises your pulse rate, reddens your face with upset and raises your anger levels, you rather don't get involved in such situations.

Try and express feelings instead of bottling them up. If someone or something insults you, express your feelings frankly. Don't bottle them up. If you express your feelings openly, it could be that you will prevent a build up resentments that will preserve negative feelings and frustration.

Re-definition of the situation that causes stress. Try and find positive aspects in the situation. This is an opportunity to see things from a positive perspective. Could it be that something positive will come out of this situation? Perhaps dealing with this stressful occurrence will lead to personal growth? Or perhaps this challenge will lead to improved skills to handle future difficulties.

Perspective of time. Try to see yourself in the future, foreword in three or ten years. How will this annoying situation look in a long term perspective? What will you think of how you behaved today? Was it worth all the stress and annoyance? Was it really worth losing your balance? Perhaps it would have been better to preserve your energy for better more constructive things.

When we look at things from a future perspective we get a completely different view. We see ourselves in a wider, more general picture.

Perfectionism- Sometimes, when our minimum is only complete perfection, and we are never satisfied with less, it is very easy to fail. Failure is the root of a lot of stress. One can easily get rid of this stressor by lowering our aspirations.

Sometimes an average result is okay. Nothing will happen if things are not perfect. This understanding can prevent failure that can lead to unnecessary pressure and stress.

Learn to focus on the positive. Even when you are in a stressful situation that you can't change, you can consider the positive aspects of your life. What you have within you, things you did successfully, perhaps more than others. When we train ourselves to look at positive aspects of our life, to always see the half full cup and not half empty! And we focus on things like a stable marriage, children, home and job, and then the stressful events will be less significant.

Learn to forgive. For as long as we cannot learn to forgive others, we will be storing anger and resentment inside us. The only ones who are hurt by this bottling up of resentment are us. This negative emotional energy can be extremely destructive and can lead to long-term physical and mental damage. Holding on to resentment keeps us from replenishing positive feelings that we spread around us. This step will allow us to move on to a better, more positive place and to use our energy for useful and constructive purposes.

Don't try to be in control of an uncontrollable situation. Learn to let go! How many times have we tried and failed to take control of life events? How many times have we tried to change something that cannot be changed? Should we waste our strength for nothing in a place that we have no influence? The ability to let go of resentments are learned skills that can really lower our frustration levels.

Strengthen your relations with friends and family-Many people feel alone and isolated from society. This can cause them anxiety. They can turn to look for virtual relations. In this way the addicted person develops a completely different character from his usual self. Strengthening the connection with family, parents, spouses and children will do a lot to relieve loneliness and the fear of being alone.

Your Life is in Your Own Hands Take Responsibility

Be your own manager.

In the previous chapter, we showed a lot of factors that impact the causes of internet addiction.

This includes Negative feelings, low self and social esteem, bad experiences, the need to be accepted a need to be part of a social group to get a feeling of belonging, looking for excitement and thrills. All these are powerful factors that work in the background and can cause us to be trapped into addiction. You lose control and cannot stop the downward spiral. All addictions cause suffering and a feeling of frustration, shame and guilt. Something is controlling you. You are not the boss of your own life.

The link between negative feelings and addiction is clear and proven. Usually it is emotional pain that is largely catalyzing the addiction.

What feds negative feelings? Usually it is the system of basic beliefs that we have about ourselves. These lead to negative self-talk that express these beliefs like "I'm worthless!", "Nobody likes me", "I look strange", "I'm all alone." These basic self-concepts have a big influence over the way we manage our feelings. When emotional management is conducted efficiently, it is much easier to manage the addiction.

When these basic self-concepts and thought patterns are in order, the person will feel balanced and will be able to manage himself effectively.

Our aim is to gain control over the source of the addiction and from this point it will be easier to control ourselves and our internet surfing habits. The self beliefs are the way a person perceives himself even though he may not always be consciously aware of these beliefs. Like deep-flowing underground water, these self-beliefs are penetrating deep into our life. Sometimes these self beliefs are taken as completely true but in fact they are not at all. If you get to know your own self-beliefs, it will be easier to see if they are true and how strong they are.

You may have to adapt a more constructive and realistic self-image.

Examples of basic self-beliefs

I am not socially accepted.

I will never succeed socially.

I can't control myself.

I'm alone.

I'm damaged.

I'm rejected.

I'll never succeed in life.

I'm worthless.

I'm unwanted.

I'm a bad person.

I'm a failure.

I'm different.

I don't deserve love.

No-one loves me.

I can't do anything properly.

The world is not a safe place.

I'm very sensitive.

I'm ugly.

Somehow we believe that these self beliefs are true although they are completely not true. The problem with these concepts is that they can motivate us to act in a negative way.

Once we have a clear understanding about what in fact is guiding us in a large part of our thinking and behavior patterns, we will have a better chance to minimize their influence on our lives.

Ron was introverted person for as long as he could remember himself. Since he was a child he believed he would never be socially accepted. The thought: "I am not accepted" was very prominent in his mind. It was a kind of social anxiety.

When he discovered the social networks on the internet, he began to spend more and more time in the chat-rooms. Slowly Ron detached himself from everything in his life and spent all his nights in on-line interactions. He was fired from his job since he missed a lot of hours each day.

His frustration caused him to sink deeper into addiction and he spent most of his days on the internet, using the social networks. In this way Ron was trying to deal with his self-belief that he would never be successful in social relations. He tried again and again to prove to himself that he was able to connect to people by the internet. Finally A friend referred him to a therapist who specialized in addiction. Here he began his path of admitting that he had a problem. This process also included working on his self concepts and negative thought patterns. Ron came to understand that his self belief was standing in his way and it had become a self-fulfilling prophesy. Gradually he returned to a normative lifestyle and he got a better job than he had before. Today, Ron is a volunteer in a support group to help other addicted people.

Emotional self management is a key factor in a person's control over internet surfing habits. Feelings are often a result of the interpretation that you give to events. If we understand the situation correctly, the feelings that arise will be manageable. But when our interpretation is overblown, the emotion is stirred up.

The emotional distress that comes about is fertile ground for an addiction to arise. Some addicts were exposed for negative environment in their childhood. They experienced humiliation and rejection. These circumstances naturally cause long internal distress and inner pain. Many of them have life problems like difficult relationships, unemployment, health issues, emotional instability, a low motivation for change and feelings of hopelessness.

It doesn't mean that each one of these problems is what has caused the addiction or fuels it, but it could be that the problem was a factor in getting to this point.

When we develop mistaken self-concepts, it might lead us in a wrong way to mechanism of compensation. This can lead us to addictive, maladaptive behavior.

On this distorted self beliefs, we will create thoughts, feelings and behavior that can lead to addiction. When an addictive style of thinking overtakes us, we look at the world through completely different lenses and this mistaken perception change the way we see things.

Because we are not conscious of this pattern, we come to the conclusion that we have to find an escape, a secure area where it will be easier to cope. This way, we are repeatedly trapped in the same negative cycle where running away from reality increases our problems twice as much. Our job is to break this bubble of illusion, to look in to ourselves and at what caused us to run away to an imaginary refuge. We need to find the root of our feelings, examine how we deal with them, and pinpoint the mistaken beliefs about ourselves and the negative thought patterns that lead to them.

In order to understand how we get in to negative emotional states, we must understand what stands at the base of the thoughts that led us into such negative feelings.

Remember: Thoughts lead to feelings!

Not only does thought *come before* feeling, thought *creates* feelings.

Remember the model:

Event- Interpretation- Feeling-reaction

The event affects our thoughts that in turn cause feelings and this leads to the reaction.

Identifying automatic thoughts is important factor in gaining emotional control. The more you practice identifying your negative thoughts, the more you will improve your ability to control them, and put them in their right perspective.

We tend to believe that the automatic thoughts that stream in our heads are the absolute truth when this is not the case at all.

We don't always test the accuracy of our thoughts.

Our automatic thoughts tend sometimes to catastrophe. They see danger and dark at every opportunity and always foresee the worst. In this way, small ache can be a terrible disease. When these thoughts come up, there is a tendency to exaggerate the severity of the situation. This can lead to anxiety. These automatic thought usually focus on failures and flaws, on negative events, or on the past. They cause us to look only at one aspect of the situation, usually a negative aspect, and ignore all the rest.

Negative thoughts usually include cognitive distortions.

We will get to know them:

Ten Cognitive Distortions

Thought distortions are extremely powerful. Dr David barns described them in his book "feeling good" They work on an unconscious level and their influence on our thoughts and feelings is very strong.

everything or nothing! (perfectionism)- trying to run after absolute completeness. Any result that is less than perfect causes a person to feel worthless. Usually it is impossible to uphold these expectations in the long term and the result is a feeling of failure, disappointment and low self-esteem. Perfectionism sets an impossibly high standard for success and when the person does not attain this standard, the feeling is of a complete downfall.

Overgeneralization-The occurrence of a single event gives the feeling that from here on, this is what will always happen. A single personal episode becomes something general and fundamental. For example, my husband came in to the house and didn't smile at me, so apparently, from now on, he won't love me anymore.

A mental filter- this is an unconscious pattern. Positive or neutral experiences are perceived negatively. It is usually the attempt to constantly prove to yourself that you are not good enough or you are defective in some way.

It expresses itself in a lack of ability to enjoy good moments in life. It leads to an unnecessary feeling of misery.

Jumping to conclusions mind reading. This is attempt to judge or try to guess what other people are thinking or feeling about you. It is trying to "prophesize" what the other person is thinking about you and to draw conclusions. This mind-reading seems very logical at the time and the person is sure they have reached the correct conclusion and what they think is in fact, true.

Future telling This is the type of pessimistic view that looks at the future as if it has already happened and the future events have already happened and are an irreversible fact.

Disqualifying the positive-Taking positive or neutral experiences and turning them in to bad experiences. The positive aspects are not only ignored, but turned into negatives. All the good parts of the experience are filtered out and the negative sides are emphasized.

Catastrophic thinking- Every small thing becomes an unbearable catastrophe. This catastrophic imagination is unlimited and leads to a terrible feeling that something terrible is about to happen. This kind of thinking leads to deep pessimism and a dark outlook.

Magnification and minimization- There are glasses that can magnify or diminish size. Similarly, there are thought distortions that exaggerate the importance of mistakes, or events.

Personalization- Creating a negative personal image because of mistakes. Looking in a negative way on people. This causes us to develop hostility towards them.

It is very important to differentiate between your actions and the essence of yourself as a person. When a person builds a negative identity for himself, based on something negative he did, he is likely to have feelings of guilt and worthlessness.

"Should" and "must" statements:

Saying "I must" or "I have to" are a high standard that you set for yourself. When you do not manage to achieve this result, you feel self hate, shame and feelings of guilt, as well as other negative feelings. These inner instructions like "I have to" and "i must" cause pressure and resentment. These words of "have to" and "must" can also be directed at others,

"He needs to do this," and "She has to do that." And this causes a lot of frustrated feelings. You feel that you have to behave a certain way, but you don't check objectively if you are making a logical demand of yourself. This thought pattern causes mental rigidity, sticking to mistaken basic premises and criticizing yourself and others.

Personal responsibility- taking responsibility for negative situations even when they have nothing to do with me. This is the tendency to see everything going on around us as being our fault. An example for this is a husband who interprets his wife's comments on how expensive everything is in the shops as an attack on his ability to earn a living. This thought distortion causes feelings of blame and guilt as a result of taking heavy responsibility on oneself.

One needs to be aware that other people's actions are their responsibility. They chose to do these acts and only they can be responsible for them.

All these thought distortions can cause us unpleasant feelings. A large range of negative feelings and emotional distress can develop as a result of these distortions.

These can be anxiety, phobias, and feelings of shame, negative self-image and even depression in all its degrees. It is very important to get to know these negative thought patterns so we can isolate them and deal with them properly.

The Triple Column Technique

This technique was developed by Dr. David Barns. How can we get rid of these cognitive distortions and their destructive emotional results?

First we have to get to know them well and identify them when we come across them every day. With time we will learn that this negative self-talk is not always a reflection of reality. Putting doubt about these thoughts in our own minds is an important stage in dealing with them. Gradually, the difficult feelings that comes as a result from this thoughts will also diminish. In order to cope with this problem we have to deal with its roots. These are the self-beliefs and negative self talk that comes with them. The technique we use is the Triple Column Technique.

We write down these automatic thoughts. Than we try to practice exchanging this thoughts with thoughts that are objective facts.

Automatic Thoughts (Self-Criticism)	Cognitive Distortion	Rational response (self-defense)
I can't live without the internet	generalization	There were times in my life that I lived without the internet and I was perfectly fine!
I have difficulties I have to surf the net to feel better.	generalization	I can deal with difficulties using other methods. Overusing the internet is not a

		compensation but a problem on its own!
I am a weak person. I can't fight my internet addiction.	Labeling Fortune-telling/ seeing the future	I'm not so weak. That's not true. In many areas I am strong. With the right help I will overcome this addiction.
My friends will mock me if I'm not online in the chat room. They won't understand why I'm cutting	Mind-reading/	Maybe someone will be disappointed but that's not a tragedy. My life is more important than what others think of me.

myself off.		

Did you notice what happened here? We took automatic thoughts that we have never evaluated before, that cause us negative feelings. We checked their validity and we gradually reduce the influence that negative thoughts have over us. We recognize exaggerated self-criticism that we direct at ourselves and we put it in proportion.

Table of Events and a Declaration of Coping Strategies

We can use a similar technique for events that bother us. It can be a past event or something that happens to us from time to time. The rule is not to let automatic thoughts take control of us and cause us negative feelings. We can defend ourselves against these thoughts in a rational way, and thus decrease their influence.

Sometimes an answer to these automatic thoughts is not enough. We need to make a declaration of the fact that we are going to cope with the situation and deal with it actively. We will stand up to it in an effective way.

This declaration of coping helps us to counteract the fear that we have of the event. It gives us encouragement and power to leave this event with added strength. Below is a table of events and possible declarations of coping.

Event	Threat Level- What is the possibility that something will happen?	The first thought that comes in to our heads.	Declaration of coping

Examples of Declarations of coping

1. This is an unpleasant feeling but I can stand it. I will manage myself and my feelings.

2. Many people have coped with the same situation before me and managed. There's no reason why I can't do the same.

3. There are always difficulties. The thing is to deal with them.

4. I will not let outside events control me.

5. I don't want to be controlled by others.

6. I won't die because of this. In the end it will pass.

7. Just because I feel this way doesn't mean that it's true. Feelings are not facts.

8. I won't let others push me off balance.

9. I'm choosing to cope with it.

10. My own interpretation is not the right one.

The table allows us to move from the point we are controlled by the fear of the event to a place where we cope with the event and control our feelings and manage them.

Listening to Myself

In this method we will practice examining these thoughts without being critical and judicial.

Look at your thoughts from the side, as if you are a man standing on the edge of the river and looking at leaves and bits of wood floating by in the water. The leaves simply float on by.

Just the fact that you are looking in to your flow of thoughts at a given time without being judicial will allow you to control these thoughts flowing through your mind and to supervise their content.

The issues that need special attention are:

1. To be aware of our continual stream of consciousness. Observe this flow of thoughts without being judicial or critical.

2. To identify negative thoughts that come up from time to time and to be doubtful about the truth of what they imply.

3. To try and get used to a more rational attitude instead of negative self-talk with its criticism and judgmental attitude to ourselves and others. Change your internal dialogue to something more positive.

This self-talk that influences our feelings so much can be changed. Self talk should not be negative and critical but should help you reach important goals in your life more quickly.

Do you really want to change?

For most of us, the word "change" sounds good. Actually, making a change demands a huge amount of effort and energy.

In order to begin the process of change, it is important to get to know the main components of this process.

Pre-contemplation Stage:

At this stage you are not yet aware that there is a problem. Internet surfing habits are out of control, and there is no sign that you want to change the way things are. At this stage there is no taking of personal responsibility.

You are controlled by the addiction and you don't have the tools to deal with it.

In order to escape the problem you have to understand the losses you have by staying with the addiction.

Rumination: (Thinking about Change)

At this stage you are already more aware of the problem and you do have a will to treat it. Being addicted engages your thoughts and bothers you. You don't believe that you will ever be able to do it to overcome the addiction. This stage of rumination can either be very short or can take few years!

Decision:

At this stage there are already practical decisions being made about what steps need to be taken to solve the problem. Usually this stage will action needed to be taken and fund-raising needed to put the plan in to practice.

Action:

At this stage perhaps you are making attempts to stop the addiction by yourself. These attempts usually fail. You look for information and ask others for help. If you reach the right places, then you will begin a steady process of rehabilitation. With proper support you will successfully leave the addiction behind you.

Preservation: (Keeping up the good work!)

This stage is perhaps the most important. We will attempt to preserve the progress we have made and keep up the good work. At this stage it is worthwhile to keep adding tools that will help us to cope so we can carry on with the effort to stay clean from addiction.

Regression:

It could be that even with all the efforts we made to keep up the good work, there will still be a regression and we will slide back into addiction. We must remember that a falling is not a failure. This dynamic will move the process forward right from the start. At the second time round you will have been strengthened by the experience.

Now you will have to go back to the starting point and from there, try to get to a level that you will be able to uphold in a more permanent way. Every change always has its ups and downs. So if you slip up, you should see it as a way to strengthen yourself for continuing the process.

These are the steps of the change. Now ask yourself: Where are you on the list? Are you thinking about change?

You're progressing!

The fact that you're reading this book means that you've made an important step in the direction of a real change and you have an excellent chance to climb all the way up.

Have you already reached the stage where you have made a decision?

When you **choose** to decide, you will have a crucial influence over your addiction to the internet.

Emotional management

In many cases, internet addiction developed because a person got caught in negative feelings that brought him to emotional pressure. This feeling of relief made by surfing the internet carry on until he was out of control and addicted. How did he get into such a state?

When we deal with negative feelings that can bring us to addictive behavior, the key to success is a proper emotional management. When our interpretation of events is extreme and does not match actual events, then abnormal feelings are very hard to deal with. The emotional distress that results can give a push to the addiction.

Humiliation and rejection cause inner pain and real distress. There are many addicts who were subjected to negative treatment from their environment that was traumatic for them. There are many addicts who have hard lives. Some of them are unemployed, and this causes feelings of worthlessness and anxiety about how they will exist and support their families. Some of them have health problems or difficult family relationships. Some of the addicts suffer from emotional instability. It is a matter of survival to manage feelings properly. Some of them just think they can never change, perhaps because they feel hopeless or have a low motivation to change. It doesn't mean that any one of these problems is what fuels the addiction or caused it. But it is likely that there are few factors that have pushed them over the edge.

Gad, a high-school student had mistaken basic beliefs about himself that he was worthless and not successful. He used computer games as a compensatory mechanism. His emotional turmoil and the feeling "I'm nothing!" led him to addictive, maladaptive behavior Based on mistaken self-beliefs. Soon he realized that these beliefs hurt him. Then he met a psychologist that helped him get out of the problem.

Every one of us builds whole buildings of thoughts, feelings and behavior that can lead us to look for something that will compensate us, like the internet. We get to a point where an addictive style of thinking overtakes us. Reality looks very different through this lens. We lock ourselves into a certain way of thinking and don't give room to any other view. Caught in a pattern that we are not even aware of, we reach the conclusion that we have to escape! To find a refuge! Where will we find a safe place that will relieve our distress? In this way we get caught up again and again in that same negative cycle that any attempt to escape leads us deeper in to the mud, and the situation gets worse and worse.

If Gad would have looked in to himself, he would have identified the negative feelings that caused him to look for an imaginary, exciting refuge. He would have been able to examine the roots of the feelings that struck him and would have been able to deal with them in a constructive, useful way. We have to burst the bubble of self-deceit and to find our mistaken self-beliefs and the negative thought patterns that lead us in to addiction.

Once we have identified these mistaken basic beliefs and destructive thought patterns, it will be easier to build new self-concepts and to exchange our thought patterns for more beneficial ones. This way we will come to more positive feelings and an inner balance.

Developing emotional intelligence and correct management of feelings is very important if we don't want to act like robots automatically using old, familiar patterns that we developed over the years.

Some of us developed problematic behavior patterns like impulsivity, irritability, anger, a tendency to be pressured from every little thing and more. Is this the correct, gainful choice right now? Does this choice really let me progress or is it damaging? Will this help me in the future?

Managing emotions is a learned skill. We are able to learn how to fit our feelings into the area of personal choice. Not unconscious, automatic management, but bringing about feelings as a result of choice and self awareness. For that reason we need to know ourselves and the patterns by which we act. It could be that these patterns are stumbling blocks that trap us without being aware of it.

We sometimes find ourselves reacting automatically with an angry attack, fear, aggression. These are only a few of the patterns that are so difficult to get away from. When we empower our self awareness and highlight these feelings, we will gradually be able to control them more and more.

The most important thing is that our reactions should come from a personal choice.

Imagine an event where you are about to park your car, and suddenly another car pushes into your space. You could be annoyed or angry. Perhaps you'd shout or even insult the driver.

What was the dynamic here? You were controlled and mannered by others.

You were not in control of yourself. When we are not in control of ourselves, we are controlled by other factors and then we have a problem.

What exactly is happening here? Perhaps it is our personal interpretation? Maybe he didn't see us? Did you perhaps think about the fact that it wasn't worth losing control like that?

Most anger comes from personal interpretation and not from the actual event. In any case our choice has to be that we control our feelings and not allow anyone else to control us.

When we learn how to manage our feelings in the right way, we will use them to strengthen our inner sense of well being and happiness. our feelings will not take us anymore to places of frustration and negative feelings that can push us further and deeper into addiction and uncontrolled, obsessive internet use. When we are managing our feelings, we won't be controlled by events and people and we won't get stuck with the unwelcome results that can come out of it. Then, without a doubt, our life will be free from resentments and anger.

What Can We Do To Overcome Addiction?

Many of us have tried to stop out-of-control internet surfing and failed. Feelings of guilt shame, humiliation and worthlessness. These are only some of the emotions that we feel when we are trapped in the vicious cycle of internet addiction.

So what will help us to actually solve the problem?

First of all we need to admit to ourselves that we have lost control over our internet surfing habits. This admission and awareness helps us to progress in the direction of finding a solution.

Finding and identifying our uncontrolled patterns will help us be more aware of the problem and its background causes.

Has it ever happened to you that you planned to sit for half an hour near the computer and the time stretched to three or four hours? Do you lose your sense of time passing when you are using the internet?

Is it difficult to get you to move away from the computer when you are online?

Are you waiting impatiently to get back on-line while you are busy with other things?

Getting to know the signs of addiction in internet use will help us to be aware of it when we come across these signs in real time.

The most outstanding characteristic of addiction is a loss of control. The addicted person is in a whirlpool that sucks him deeper and deeper and he cannot overcome the urge to surf the net and go to sites that express his addiction. These can be gaming sites; gambling sites pornography sites on-line casinos, chat rooms, social networks, and more.

Before we begin with the techniques in this chapter, it would be useful to get away from the net to a place where you will not use the computer at all.

This can be done by going on a trip, or a vacation where you will take care to completely be free of internet usage.

After a complete break of at least a week, putting the techniques in this chapter will be much easier. This break is extremely helpful.

Nevertheless, even if you are not able to take a holiday, or incapable of cutting yourself off, don't give up the idea!

It is possible to make these steps even without the break.

Tracking log

Every day write down the amount of hours you surf on the net and what sites you go to. Use a special diary that you have assigned for this purpose. This will enable you to track your internet habits. It will increase your awareness of yourself and what you do in real time.

Take special note to which sites you are attracted. it is very important for the next step.

Write down what are the situations and triggers that bring you to sit down in front of the computer. Perhaps it is a disappointment you had today that made you frustrated? Did someone hurt you or get angry with you and made you upset? Is it a feeling of inner emptiness that bothers you?

Sometimes we can identify a situation that happens over and over that repeatedly pushes us to seek escape in prolonged internet usage.

Finding the situation or the frustrating relationship that cause us to run away and hide on the net is very important. It enables us to neutralize this urge when we come across it again.

C.B.T. Cognitive Behavioral Therapy

This technique allows one to neutralize the obsession and negative patterns behind internet usage.

If there are additional problems in the background like depression or anxiety that empower the obsessive internet surfing, this technique will also be very effective.

With this method, we identify negative thought patterns that contribute to the creation of negative feelings. These, in their turn, feed anxiety and depression. This method brings us better self awareness regarding the forces that influence us and provide ways to neutralize them.

Filtering and Blocking

Filtration from your internet provider that blocks unsuitable internet sites has a crucial importance. Many internet suppliers provide their subscribers with filters. One should take advantage of these to block any possibility of getting to sites of dubious content. In a house where there are children such a filter is necessary. Filtered internet access is likely to prevent many of the dangers on the net.

Parental control programs can be a very useful means of protection if you cannot be there to supervise your children's use of the internet or you are far from home. There are parents who hide the existence of this tracking program from their children and some of them notify their kids that there is such a program in place on the computer so they will not try anyway to get to any unsuitable sites. You will have to decide what the best approach for your family.

A Balance of Profit and Loss

When the owner of a business balances his income and expenses, he can see exactly how profitable his business is. Contrasting the advantages and disadvantages of obsessive internet usage by writing it down on paper or in chart form in an organized fashion can be an important step in developing awareness and control over internet surfing habits.

Make a chart:

On one side, write the advantages you have from your internet usage. On the other side write the disadvantages: the losses you sustain as a result of your internet usage and their direct and indirect influence on your life.

This can be how it influences your work; your relationships you have with your children, your spouse; your social life.

Reading this chart from time to time and updating it makes us progress and awaken in to a deeper awareness. This in time will lead us to action and better control over our internet surfing habits.

It is important that you define to yourself and make a distinction as to what is absolutely necessary use of the internet like work needs, or study, and how much time is spent for it or out of control surfing. This second sort enslaves us and leads us to neglect all other areas of our lives if.

This distinction will help to make the time you spend on the internet more efficient.

Using the internet may be part of your life because you need it for your job or to be in contact with your family.

Surfing becomes a problem when we ignore spouses and family and the fact that we need to invest in them emotionally.

If we are not able to stop even though we can see that there are negative effects on our life, this is the time to handle the problem.

Is it really worth

Obsessive Internet Surfing	Moderate, Normative Internet Surfing
Feelings of depression, anxiety and guilt.	Strengthening self-confidence and positive feeling.
Parents and family are angry with me.	Family and friends are happier with me.
My work has dropped. Also my income.	My work has improved, also my income.
I am not in control of myself; I am	I control my own life. Nothing controls me.

controlled by my addiction.	
I am missing out on and wasting real life. My life is spent in a virtual bubble.	I live in the real world. I have real relationships.
I don't deal with real problems in life because I'm busy with my addiction.	I can deal with urgent problems in my life and find solutions for them.
A terrible waste of time. I could be doing good things during this time.	I have free time to do the things I've always wanted to do, and couldn't.

Support Groups

Joining support groups is a very common way of seeking support. One can find these groups that provide support for almost any subject.

It is important to join a support group whose members are dealing with the same problem that you are in order to get new strength. This way we feel that we are not alone.

Usually, groups that deal with addiction use the 12 Steps Program to enable rehabilitation. This technique was originally developed for alcoholics but it is effective for all types of addiction.

The main benefits of a group are breaking down the isolation that so much characterizes the addict, and providing tools for dealing with the addiction. These tools help to cope with difficulties and frustration, and raise the addicted person's self-worth.

Above all, these groups and this path allow him to progress along a well-traveled safe route that is true for helping people cope with their addiction. Some of the things that one learns in a group are how to put off perpetual dissatisfaction, becoming one and linking to a Higher Power that can help us by giving us strength to face the challenge and to deal with the difficulties that brought us to this situation. The group also guides one how to keep on with the good work once the addiction has been left behind.

The members of the group reflect parts of our character that we can't see for ourselves. Group members help each other and share experiences and feelings. The more frank the members of the group are with each other, and open to sharing, the more they will gain from the rehabilitation process.

Part of the task is revealing feelings. This is not always easy but it is an important move that leads to great progress.

A person addicted to the internet sometimes develops a virtual character that is completely different from his real personality. With the help of the people in the group, we can see how we look in the eyes of the real world as is reflected in the way the group sees us.

For a long time, the internet addiction hide the truth about us. Now we are learning how to experience the real world and real relationships.

The 12 Step Program

The Twelve Step program was developed by Alcoholics Anonymous and was put in to practice also by other rehabilitation groups like O.A. (Overeaters Anonymous, G. A. (Gamblers Anonymous), N.A. (Narcotics Anonymous). In this program the addiction is described as a disease. By carrying out the steps of this program, one can recover.

Personal will is not enough to leave the problem behind. Addiction is not something that can be beaten by willpower alone. Those who tried to stop their addiction using only their own willpower failed time after time. We start with admitting that the problem is out of control and we are helplessness in the face of trying to control it.

Admitting that we are helplessness is the point from where we start to recover. Only from this specific point can progress on the path to overcoming the problem take place. This is the first step on that path. From this point of our realization of our own helplessness against our addiction, we can give up the attitude of fighting against the disease with our own strength and we give ourselves over to a Higher Power, the power of G-d. Only this way can we get real help, only He has the power to release us from the craving and the non-stop urge to surf the internet.

It could be that we made attempts in the past to stop by ourselves but because we never asked for help, these attempts were always a failure.

Here we directly fight the problem. We admit that we have lost control over our lives because of the addiction and we ask someone stronger than us for help. Perhaps this step seems like a weak, fearful reaction, but in fact it is the strongest action. Admitting that there is a problem stronger than we are.

From here on we start strengthening ourselves and building up a new positive personal identity.

Submission means that we understand that all the ways we tried till now have failed and we need a new, different way to overcome the problem. This submission also means that we know we can't control the problem by ourselves and we are actually powerless in the face of it and we need the help of a Higher Power to overcome it.

Giving ourselves over in to the hands of a Higher Power is one of the basic ideas of the 12 Steps. When we are bound with something above us which is limitless and incomparably greater and stronger than us, we get new strength and we are able to deal with our addiction. This can be compared to a dwarf standing on the shoulders of a giant.

Because he is on the giant he can see farther into the distance. We learn how to put ourselves into the hands of a Higher Power and to ask for help to overcome the cravings or any other difficulties that threaten to push us back into addiction.

The 12 Step Program is not meant only to put us on the road to recovery. It also gives us tools for a life of satisfaction and meaning.

As was stated above, the process of this program leads us to link up with something bigger than ourselves.

This can also be understood in a different, more limited way. This bigger and stronger power could be the group effect, an objective friend who we share with, professional advice and more. All these factors can give us new strength to deal with the addiction. Usually, each addicted person finds a sponsor who guides him through the process. Keeping in touch with this sponsor is very important, especially in the first stages, when the urge to go back to the addiction is the strongest. One of the ways of overcoming powerful craving is to phone your sponsor and talk. A conversation like this can ease the difficulty and even banish it.

The group program puts the 12 steps into practice.

The first step is admitting the problem is stronger than us. or as the group proclaims: "We admitted that we were powerless over the addiction, that we lost control over our lives."

The other steps include recognizing that help comes from a Higher Power that can rescue us from this problem. Then there is a searching and fearless moral inventory, atoning for past actions, a spiritual awakening that comes as a result of a conscious contact with a Higher Power and giving over the message to others addicts.

It is basically a program of spiritual growth. Going through the steps of the program allows a person to grow spiritually. We make a fundamental change in the way we look at things and at the significant relationships in our life.

Emotional release

One of the problems linked with internet addiction is a proper management of feelings.

Negative feelings urge us to find an escape, any port in a storm. They can drag us to places that we don't want. These places may seem like they will help us deal with our inner pain. The addiction usually feeds off inner distress that follows us through our lives. This distress can come about for a number of reasons. like a feeling of inner emptiness and meaninglessness, frustration over relationships with family and friends, problems at work, a negative emotional load from the past or childhood or problems that can't be solved. All these are only part of a wide spectrum of situations that can lead to emotional distress.

There are some techniques that can diffuse negative emotional distress. Some of these will do so by invoking feelings and talking about them. This brings them up and into our conscious minds. Then we can take apart these emotions and deal with them.

Some use N. L. P. (Neuro-Linguistic Programming) to reach the same goals.

You need to find the way that is most suitable for you and that you feel you can connect with to remove negative feelings caused by your own personal circumstances.

Dismantling negative feelings like anxiety, anger and frustration is a very important step on the way to achieving inner stability. When we are emotionally stable and feel good within ourselves, it is easier for us to deal with addiction.

Time Management

Time management is a skill that can be learned. Even if we are not born with this ability, we can develop it. We can plan our day and what we will do in every part of it. We will decide of a certain, limited amount of time that we can be in front of the computer.

It is clear that we will define a time for ourselves that we need to finish our tasks without deviating from them in the middle. The rule here is to develop awareness in real time to what is happening to us and developing personal responsibility for managing our time right. One of the most important points of time management is setting a time to go to sleep. If we know that we need seven hours of sleep, we will plan our time so that the body will get the rest it needs.

When we plan our time, we are aware of what happens to us on a time scale, and it is much easier to be aware of obsessive internet surfing where we lose all sense of time.

A Meaningful Life

Meaninglessness, a feeling of emptiness is some of the feelings that can affect people these days.

Here the opportunity rises up to look for thrills that will compensate this emptiness.

Many people who are addicted to the internet say about themselves that they feel that their lives are shallow and lacking content.

Obsessive surfing of the net is like a screen that covers over the sad truth, their emptiness and boredom.

One of the important basics of the 12 Step Program for rehabilitation from addiction is pouring spiritual content and experience into ones life and connecting to a Higher Power. When a person lives connected to a Higher Power, it helps him to stay clean. This way he does not have to run after thrills and immediate satisfaction. This constant search for thrills is linked to the experience of inner lack. Something is missing, and we try to balance it out with thrill-seeking and excitement.

Paradoxically, running after thrills and excitement only strengthens and amplifies our negative feelings.

Giving ourselves over to a Higher Power comes in to play. This is a very important aspect of rehabilitation.

Giving ourselves over to a Higher Power allows us to begin a more satisfying life and allows us to get strength to stay free of addiction.

The importance of a transition to a life of meaning is crucial. Looking for thrills comes from boredom and emptiness. Learn to fill yourself with new, spiritual content.

When we strive for a life full of meaning and connection to G-d, we will get a new, fresh strength that will help us to stay clean from addiction.

Running Away or Coping?

Have you ever thought about the fact that internet addiction is a kind of running away to a virtual world where the rules of coping with a situation are different than those in the real world?

This escape to a virtual world can cause great difficulty when we want to come back to the real world.

Illusion and reality are mixed up together in our minds and as a result of this, problems come up in our day to day function.

The virtual identity causes us to live a double life. Virtual characters prevent us from improving our real self. Usually there is a connection between developing a virtual character and not accepting oneself, or low self esteem. When it is hard to accept ourselves and our self-image is negative, the tendency to look for or to build a new, illusory self that will compensate us and give us positive value in our own eyes and in the eyes of others.

In this case, one needs to go through a process of personal empowerment, to build up a positive self image and to be accepting of oneself without being judicial.

Perpetual dissatisfaction

Many people live with a sense of dissatisfaction in their lives.

There is a feeling of a terrible waste of strength and talents. Addicted person levels of dissatisfaction are much higher than usual. This feeling causes disquiet and a desire to look for some sort of compensation that will relieve the bad feelings. We can compare this to trying to fill a barrel that has a hole in it. All attempts to fill it up will fail. We will always have to add more and more. All attempts will fail. There are some people who have this bottomless, feeling of emptiness. There is never a sense of true satisfaction. There is always a craving to find new excitement. This constant dissatisfaction can lead us into unexpected places and situations.

On the other hand, if we choose to cut ourselves off from this dependence on outside satisfaction and to understand that there is no way that we will get to real happiness when we are in a state of dependence; we take a step in the right direction. The type of satisfaction does not matter. If we understand this then it will be easier for us to deal with our addiction.

In fact, every moment we have the perpetual choice: To deal with the difficulty or to run away from it.

When we cope with difficulties at home, at school or at work, we are moving towards growth and development. When we choose to run away from problems because we are anxious or because it makes us uncomfortable, things get even worse. Usually we try to escape by looking for something that will make us feel better.

Running away from our own difficulties causes them to come up even stronger.

This is what happens when we use the internet obsessively. We do so in order to cope in ineffective way with our inner discomfort. When we come to understand that this pattern of running away that we have adopted only makes things much worse, it will be easier to move forward from this point.

Normal, moderate use of the internet is okay. This is not like other addictions (like alcohol or drugs) that demand complete abstinence. In this case, a complete break is not necessary, but you have to control your time, and be constantly on guard against obsessive surfing.

Personal Growth

In order to be fully rehabilitated from addiction, we need to treat not only the negative elements that influence us but we also need to start on a process of personal growth. We need to be willing to profound change in the way we manage our thoughts and feelings in order to achieve personal growth. The choice to make a change is in our own hands. Some people claim that they don't have the strength to change their way of life. The fact we do have the power to do it.

If this is the case, why can't we do the same? The only thing that blocks a person from personal growth is he himself!

Taking down psychological barriers that keep us from personal growth is essential for fighting addiction. Rehabilitation leads us to make far-reaching, deep change in our thought patterns and the way we manage our feelings.

Self Image and Perfectionism

How do you see yourself? Do you feel that you are worth less than other people? This self-worth question is very prominent with addicts in general and with internet addicts in particular.

Mostly, we can see that addicted people suffer from a poor self image and sometimes they can't stand themselves.

A poor self-image can cause avoidance of other people in a social setting and can push the addicted person to form virtual relationships that will compensate fort the lack of real-life healthy relationships.

Understandably, low self-esteem can cause frustration and pessimistic thinking.

p.55

This is because of the thought that other people are better than him and it leads to an approach to life that is full of resentment and grievances. All these things can cause the addicted person distress and emotional pain that might cause him escaping into a virtual reality.

Sometimes we need to learn to accept ourselves and to live in peace with who we are. This doesn't mean that we don't have to make a change, but we need to know that self-acceptance is an important step tworeds making true change. If we are not able to accept ourselves, we will not be able to accept others.

The will to reach perfection in our personal lives is one of the conditions that lead to personal growth. There is, however, a different sort of perfectionism. When we think in terms of "everything or nothing" and if we did not manage 100% at everything then it means we have failed, When the standards you set is very high and you don't come up with the results you expect, there is a feeling of failure, constant dissatisfaction and negative thinking that addicted people usually suffer from.

This perfectionism can cause constant delaying of tasks or complete paralysis.

Because of our inflated expectations, we expect something so perfect that it is frightening even to begin the task. When there is a gap between the eventual result and what we expect, there is anxiety.

In order to deal with perfectionism, we need to identify the thought pattern that is "everything or nothing" in our daily functioning. Either I'm 100% or I'm nothing.

We need to be able to accept lower levels as also being success. 80% is fine!

We need to set goals for ourselves that we definitely know that are within our reach.

Social Approval

Deep in the heart of every one of us is the fear of social rejection. Of being left alone. Social relations is part of our existence, but when we start obsessing about it, and become anxious about being rejected by our social group, it can become a compulsion.

Sometimes our self esteem is completely determined by what others say about us. From this point, the road is short to becoming dependent on social acceptance where anything that threatens us with social rejection causes fear and inner anxiety. We are not talking about compliments and encouragement. Anyone is happy to get them. We are talking about a person who feels that he is "nothing" in his own right unless he gets social acceptance that will show him that he is worth something.

His self esteem and self image defend completely on what others say about him.

Ask yourself how many times you did things because of fear from social rejection.

Do you do these acts in order to get recognition from your friends?

Does your self-worth come from what others say about you?

That need for social acceptance can lead a person to lose their own identity and push them into obsessive surfing where they can get an artificial response to their needs.

The response is artificial because the affirmation that comes from these sites is aimed at the virtual character that we wish to be. Not our real identity. This affirmation and acceptance only widens the gap between the virtual character that we created and what we are in the real world.

People surfing the social networks are trying to gain the same satisfaction for the same need via the internet. This obviously causes neglecting the real-world relationships. People who are fighting for social affirmation will usually do anything to find favor in the eyes of the people around them in order to feel accepted. Their self confidence and self-worth completely depend on the opinions of others. What will happen on the day that your best friend looks angrily at you? Or someone makes a nasty comment about you?

It will bring on a feeling of worthlessness and inferiority.

This lack of stability comes from the constant dependence on social affirmation. The fear of rejection can be a factor that controls us so much that we need constantly to be told that we are part of the social group, and no-one is judging or criticizing us. Because our self-image is not strong enough, we feel the need to get ongoing reinforcement from everyone around us. This is one of the factors that can push a person towards obsessive internet surfing, the need for social affirmation.

There are some people who are online day and night on the social networks only to fulfill this need and to feel accepted and admired by other internet users. Learn to accept yourself. Learn to be able to include every part of yourself in this acceptance. Do you choose to be reliant on other people's kindness just because you need social affirmation? Your self worth is not determined by others.

When you develop a deep link with your Higher Power, with G-d, you will need less social affirmation for yourself from others. By building up your self-esteem and a positive self image that is not dependent on others, you will be more respected and esteemed by others.

We need to get the message that our self worth comes from within ourselves. I have my own inner self respect because I am a human being.

Once we realize that   , we will be free of the fear of being rejected by people and we will no longer need constant social affirmation.

Overdependence

Are you in a relationship that causes you frustration or discomfort? Is there a person that you have a relationship that causes you distress, or is there a relationship in your life that enslaves you? That you can't leave?

Do these relationships cause you the will to run away to something? Perhaps you want to make other friendships instead? Maybe being busy on the internet will compensate you for what is going on in your life?

Sometimes in order to cope with a difficulty that comes about because of over-dependency, we look for short term "solutions". These can be alcohol, overeating or internet addiction.

The common factor of these "solutions" is that they are meant to ease the pain that comes as a result of unhealthy relationships that cause stress and tension.

But like any addiction, the attempt to solve the problem in the short term by "escaping" to another place only brings new problems in the long term that are much worse than the first problem.

Sometimes the root of this behavior is in childhood. Perhaps from an emotional deficiency that came as a result of what we experienced as children. It could be negative experiences from the time of a difficult family relationship. Sometimes this behavior will come out as a result of character traits that we have.

People who are over-dependent will try and find alternative relationships on the internet in order to ease the pain they feel in the real world.

Making relationships in a real-world differs from making friends on the net.

The common ground in these uncontrolled behaviors is that they are there to cover deep, inner pain, to ease it by being obsessively busy.

People who are over-dependent stay too long in relationships that cause them mental and physical damage and emotional distress. They will be scared to take any kind of step that will anger the others and they will please them at any price. They will even compromise their basic values.

The choice is in your hands.

You can choose to spend your life in fear, frustration and self-denial. The suffering caused by such a relationship can push you in to undesirable places.

When we choose not to be controlled by fear and to free ourselves from worry we will truly free ourselves.

There is no need to rely on others only to feel we worth something. Learn to make healthy relationships that are full of love. Not relationships based on fear. Everyone deserves to be loved and it begins with the us by realizing that we deserve to be loved, and are able to give love as well.

What do you think about yourself?

What would happen if someone you know would come up to you and attack you with insults and negative opinions? You would probably answer him back, defend yourself, and try to negate what he said. You would argue with him and try to prove he is wrong.

But what happens when **you** think negative, sharp thoughts about yourself? Naturally you agree completely! It seems to you that obviously these thoughts are true! These thoughts will be interpreted by your conscious mind as if they are undeniable facts.

Why when the negative thoughts come from inside us we don't even argue with them?

The first step in dealing with the stream of negative thoughts that you have about yourself is first of all to be aware of them.

We have to be aware of the fact that these negative thoughts can become a self-fulfilling prophesy. Instead of accepting them as absolutely true, we should argue against them. We should do this with the same conviction that we would use if someone else was saying all these things about us.

We must shed doubt on these negative statements. Just the fact that we are actively questioning the truth of these thoughts will considerably minimize the effect they have on us.

Negative self-talk	Alternative thoughts
I will never be able to stop this addiction to the internet	Many people have done this before me. Why should I not succeed?
It will be terrible.	Being enslaved and

	compelled is also terrible. It will be much better if I regain control and go back to being in control of my life.
I'll go mad!	No-one ever went mad from rehabilitation.
I'll be bored. What will I do with myself?	On the contrary! I'll have lots more time to do really useful, constructive things.

Negative thoughts produce negative feelings that in their turn can make a person go in the direction of escape.

The result may be (though it doesn't have to be) looking for an available refuge.

And what is more available today if not the possibility of surfing the internet to sites that provide immediate thrills?

Isn't it preferable to choose positive thoughts that will nourish us and give us fresh strength and new energy?

The emphasis is that this is our own choice!

When we choose positive thinking we set in motion a process of change in our thoughts and inner speech.

Our personal reality is dependent on our inner speech. An old saying states that a person is where his thoughts are. We work according to our thoughts and beliefs and the results are influenced by these inner factors.

When we have a negative style of thinking: "There's no way I'll manage to get away from this!" or "I'm never going to get clear of this internet obsession!" then the results will not be encouraging.

But thoughts like: "Many people have managed to get over this, there's no reason why I won't as well!" or "I'm not worse than others who have managed, there's no reason not to try!" will stimulate me to action, and are a first, important stage in dealing successfully with the problem.

When we are focused on negative thinking, we create an atmosphere that manufactures negativity, frustration and a continuing state of addiction.

On the other hand, positive thinking will make it easier for us to break out in new directions of thought and action that will greatly increase our chances of change and recovery.

In order to adopt positive inner speech, we need to test many of our basic beliefs about ourselves that have never been tested logically.

This is especially important when we are talking about internet addiction. We have to free ourselves of constricting thoughts about ourselves. ("I'm not good, I always fail.")

Enough of this choir of devaluing voices that negates and criticizes us!

Throwing off these restrictive beliefs will help us to develop positive inner speech.

The Virtual Identity

Have you noticed that most people on social networks use nickname?

That most of the people commenting on different sites use all sorts of strange names?

Why do people on the internet build up a mask that they hide behind to conceal their real identity?

Eddie was a worker on an average salary. He was a trader on the stock market.

He presented himself on professional forums as a stock exchange professional trader with a special understanding of the stock market, and an exceptionally high success rate. Very soon he had a circle of fans on the internet who praised his analytical skills.

At the same time, Eddie's personal account was losing constantly.

His monetary losses did not prevent him from continuing presenting himself as a successful professional trader.

One fine day, there was an international incident that caused panic on the stock exchange. The world stock market fell and Eddie lost all his money. He found it very difficult to accept that he had lost everything.

It took time for Eddie to see the huge gap between the virtual character he had crafted for himself, as a successful and professional trader, and between the fact that he had a lot of loses. At the same time, the compulsive craving still beat within Eddie, causing him to sink more and more funds into the speculative buying of shares. Only when Eddie came to use the 12 Step Program in his life he started to improve and stopped gambling away his money uncontrollably.

The virtual identity created feelings of strength, power and success that he desperately needed. He loved the compliments about his brilliant analytic ability that he got on the forums. He was so entrenched in his virtual identity that he had developed that he forgot the reality. Only then he realized he had been living in a fantasy. In fact, he was very far from the virtual character he had created.

The virtual identity that Eddie created had an anesthetic effect. It strengthened his feeling that the dream of wealth was close to him. That very soon he would have a lot of money, influence and power. But actuality these feelings prevented him from dealing with the real hurtful reality, his bank account shrunk until he lost everything.

The extreme transition between the everyday identity and between the virtual identities that a person develops for himself can cause significant problems.

Managing both these identities at the same time can cause unpredictable behavior and a break with reality.

Karen was a successful teacher. After their marriage, her husband noticed that she demanded a lot of emotional response and he somehow could not keep up with her demands.

After a period of time where she used social networks on the internet she expressed her frustration over her relationship with her husband on these networks. Karen began getting emotional feedback from other men on the net.

They realized the emotional lack that she had. She used to spend whole nights on the social networks and stayed online till sunrise.

Karen began to glow. She began to feel "high".

At the beginning it was only through writing and sending messages via the internet. Soon things were out of her control and she began meeting other persons very often. Her sense of self esteem rose. She felt wanted and attractive.

The compliments she got on the social networks, like the friendships she started gave her emotional compensation for what she saw as missing in her life. She communicated with her new friends, in a way she never dared to be in real life.

Karen suddenly realized that she couldn't get herself away from what had become a twenty four hour a day obsession. She realized she was crossing red lines she had set for herself. She couldn't stop: even with these realizations.

Eventually, her husband found out about what she was doing. This caused a serious crisis in their marriage, and it almost fell apart.

In the end, Karen went through the 12 Steps Program for rehabilitation from addiction. It helped her to get back her life.

In this instance, Karen tried to build a new identity that expressed what she wanted to be:

Glowing, loved and surrounded with admiration. She created a virtual heaven for herself that was completely cut off from her reality. She drew all her self-worth from her virtual character and developed a huge dependency on social affirmation. When she came back to real life she felt she worth nothing and full of guilt and humiliation.

She learned to understand that the approvals she got from virtual relationships were empty and meaningless. Only solid relationships can give a true, satisfying connection.

The transitions between her virtual identity and between the real world were too sharp. She felt that it was hard for her to carry on keeping her secrets, and she had many of them.

The virtual identity sometimes allows a person to be aggressive and offensive because they know there will be no result. Most people who hide behind obscure identities will not be afraid to express themselves in ways that they never would dare in the real world. Many strange expressions are very common in web dialogue. The problem comes up when the transition to the real world is only partial and the virtual world overflows into the real world bringing the expressions with it.

The nickname and the virtual identity that a person adopts tell us a lot about his character. A person who calls himself by the name of a singer may identify most strongly with characters from the world of music. Someone who gives their virtual ID using the name of a world leader or a general perhaps aspires subconsciously to identify with such a figure and the power that they signify.

The virtual character demonstrates the gap and the distance between what people want to be and what they actually are in the real world. Sometimes it looks as if they build up their character to be their ideal self.

How many times we meet up with virtual characters who make themselves out to be heroes, models, politicians or army officers? characters that symbolize strength and power.

Dr. Kimberly Young, an American psychiatrist specializes in internet addiction states that very often there is a significant gap between the virtual self and the real self. The difference between the real person and the real identity can be very significant and the person has to move constantly between two worlds.

Studies show that the virtual identity influences the person's character in the real world as well.

With time, a process of adopting the traits of the virtual self into the real self comes about. This process can sometimes be negative especially when the traits adopted are negative ones like impulsivity, aggression, grandiosity etc.

Why do people build a virtual identity?

It can be explained as being an act of psychological defense. No-one likes criticism, failure and judgment.

No-one likes to be tested. The virtual identity acts as a sort of screen in order to protect us from criticism and failure.

Even if there is failure on the net it will hurt much less than if this failure had taken place in the real world. On the other hand, the success of the virtual identity is interpreted as success earned by the real identity.

But there is also another aspect. Every one of us wants to achieve self-fulfillment, and to feel that we have realized our potential. The fact is that many people live with the feeling that they have not reached self-fulfillment and that they are wasted. On the internet we can be everything. We can build a strong, powerful profile for ourselves. We can have a high level of self confidence and a good self image. No-one will say a word.

There is no hierarchy, no boss. We are not subservient to others. In our real lives we are sometimes subordinate to others and there is usually some form of hierarchy. There are rules and ethical codes that set limits. On the internet there are no limits and no barriers.

Giving power to our personal profile and the traits that we wish we had and always dreamed of, can lead to disappointment and a feeling of frustration when we come back to experience an actual relationship in the real world, because here we don't have the powerful identity that we acquired for ourselves on the internet.

The need to be linked to other people and to have social interaction also plays a major role.

Every person aspires to be socially accepted and included. The wish to be accepted socially is a deep need. When these virtual relationships develop, it is usually at the expense of real world relationships which we now neglect. As a result these real relationships degenerate over time.

When we make friends in the real world, we usually act in a polite and pleasant way, and we will try not to be aggressive. But with relationships formed on the internet, often people rid themselves of manners and act in an aggressive and impulsive way. Unexplained aggression suddenly comes to the surface. The fact that no-one really knows who we are allows us to react as if there were no barriers and without the constraint even of good manners.

This over-aggressiveness does not begin and end with the virtual interaction. Quite quickly it can burst into real world behavior. The virtual self lets us go beyond the limitations of the real world but causes problems when we want to come back to it.

This constant movement between two identities can be expressed in different ways and not all of them are constructive.

The 12 Step Program

The 12 Step Program is a way of life. It lets us progress on to a path of serenity and honesty with ourselves. The program has been created for Alcoholics Anonymous, but was later adapted to other addictions as well. Many studies show that the 12 Steps is a very effective way to cope addiction.

This is a program that combines an overall view of the addict. It is essential to go through the process in a support group. The power of a group is very important. Most of the groups are anonymous and do not demand any kind of identification. The mutual help given by the members of the group, sharing in difficulties, and being able to learn from people with experience who have gone through the process are all part of the program. It is worth to find a suitable group. There are such groups on the internet and it is easy to join them.

In order to break free from addiction we have to start with a new approach to life, stable thought patterns and emotions. This approach will help us get out of our old thinking and emotional patterns that were subconsciously feeding the addiction.

It's almost a certainty that if you have come to a decision to do something about your addiction, you must have had some serious personal difficulties. Maybe it was a family crisis with your wife or parents. Maybe there were social and financial difficulties. These significant hardships bring you to an understanding that you can't go on like this! You have to do something!

So now you have come to the point that the only way out is to grow.

This is known as the "bottom point". Every addict reaches this low point where he feels that from here on he cannot continue under any circumstances. He has to find a way out. He can't be controlled by his addiction. This bottom acts as a turning point that from here on the addict is prepared to take practical steps in order to rehabilitate himself.

The 12 Steps

1. We admitted we were powerless over our addiction, that our lives had become unmanageable.

2. Came to believe that a Power greater than ourselves could restore us to sanity.

3. Made a decision to turn over our will and our lives to the care of G-d as we understand Him.

4. Made a searching and fearless moral inventory of ourselves.

5. Admitted to G-d, to ourselves and to another human being the exact nature of our wrongs.

6. Were entirely ready to have G-d remove all these defects of character.

7. Humbly ask Him to remove our shortcomings.

8. Made a list of all persons we had harmed and become willing to make amends to them all.

9. Made direct amends to such people wherever possible except when to do so would injure them or others.

10. Continuing to take personal inventory and when we were wrong promptly admitted it.

11. Sought through prayer and meditation to improve our conscious contact with G-d   as we understood him, praying only for knowledge of His will for us and the power to carry that out.

12. Having had a spiritual awakening as a result of these Steps, we tried to carry this message to other addicts and to practice these principals in all our affairs.

Step 1: The first step begins with admitting to helplessness. Specifically when we admit that the internet addiction is stronger than us, we feel stronger than we did before. Specifically from this point, where we finally recognize that we are helpless in front of our addiction, from this point start real growth. We won't be able to control the problem with our willpower alone. This is an admission that we have no control over our addiction and it is stronger than we are. It is not always easy to admit it; our pride will sometimes make it difficult to do so.

But if we take upon ourselves to act with humility and to admit that our strength is too limited to help us in case of addiction, it will be easier to act with inner honesty.

Until today, there was denial that we had a problem, we didn't even accept the fact that we were suffering from addiction, so it was hard to admit that we were powerless against something like the internet. We had to come to the admission that the addiction is stronger than we are, and the obsessive use of the internet is controlling our life.

Have you ever felt a strong craving to go back and surf the net when you were not in front of your computer or not at home?

Have you ever been waiting for the moment when you can go and sit in front of your computer and go online? Have you ever tried to go against these urges? Do you wake up in the morning and your first thought is to run to the computer and see what's new?

The 12 Step Program demands humility from us. This humility comes in place of the denial of the problem that was before. We accept the fact that there is a problem of addiction and we try to get out of the pattern of concentrating on ourselves and our ego.

This is the opening that allows us to get help from others who have already dealt with this problem in the past. We can draw on the experiences of others who have been through this. The guidance of an experienced mentor, as well as the experience of others will make it much easier to get over the obstacles. We learn to be thankful for the positive things we have in our life (and we have them!)

To be thankful means that we learn to look at these positive things and say thank you.

Instead of the constant dissatisfaction, constant yearning that leads us to a downward spiral, we learned to acquire healthier thought patterns and to express thanks for the positive things that we have. We train ourselves to adopt a new, positive attitude and positive thought patterns by day to day thankfulness.

Every day write down five things that you are thankful for. We are looking at the positive things that we have in our life and feel satisfaction with what we have.

Step 2: In this step, we recognized that only a Power greater than us can bring us back to sane behavior. In the previous step we understood that the internet addiction is a problem that is stronger than we are. In this step, we came to understand that our own strength is not enough to overcome the problem. We won't be able to overcome the addiction on our own. By attaching ourselves to a positive, beneficent Higher Power, we can get the help we need to progress to sane behavior.

The addiction causes us to see the world through distorted glasses, and our personal judgment becomes wrong. The way we conducted ourselves was through a twisted view of the world.

Now we understand the need to connect with reality and that we have to connect to a Higher Power that can help us overcome the addiction.

Step 3: "Made a decision to turn our will and our lives over to the care of G-d as we understand Him." At this stage we are first of all deciding. We decide to choose life as our path. The power to choose is always in our hands and this has an enormous influence on the way we live our life.

We choose to utilize this power of choice in order to stop being helplessly swept away into the internet addiction. We do this consciously and with clear knowledge.

Our decision means taking responsibility. We take fresh responsibility over our lives. It is in our hands always to choose whether to walk the path of sanity, or to be swept back in to negative places and situations where we were led by addiction. Till now, we functioned by automatic patterns almost without choice.

With this step, we are first of all making a choice to choose to control our life in a way that is truly good for us.

By putting ourselves in the hands of G-d, we are linked to an eternal source of good that can help us leave the negative cycle of addiction.

Step 4: Let me introduce you to someone you've never met before- yourself!

The fourth step brings us to a deeper acquaintance with ourselves and the forces that influenced us. This is the step where we get free of a false, artificial identity and connect with our real selves. It would be very useful to write a life story in a free way. It is important to stick to the facts and less personal interpretation. we should specify the main characters in our life and how they influenced us and what was our attitude to them.

You can also write things that you've never told anyone else. At this time you don't have to reveal all of it but only to write it down. The most important thing is that writing is in itself a kind of release and intensifies self awareness. This includes getting out from resentment we have for others. During our life, we collected much resentment. These cause us feel like victims. We need to release negative energy it does not healthy to hold it. Holding on resentment can feed our emotional distress and our internet addiction.

We have to be aware of the damage that resentment brings to our life. We can stop this pain. To be caught in this distress is not something that is useful for us. The result is that the secondary damage from the constant resentment harms us much more than the original event. It could be that some of the hurts we sustained were not with intention to hurt, or that the injury was only in our own imagination.

Negative thinking is a habit that can also cause a lot of damage. Negative thought patterns can cause negative consequences in our lives. Pessimistic thinking drains our energy and leaves us emotionally emptied and more vulnerable.

Writing a fearless moral inventory about ourselves will help us to release ourselves from many negative forces that unconsciously worked against us. The more faults we uncover in ourselves, the more we will be able to continue to improve.

Step 5: This step begins with admitting to a Higher Power about the nature of our faults.
We understand that without help from this Power, we will not be able to make real progress and to become genuine and honest. With the help

of a Higher Power we leave the justifications behind us and are ready to stand face to face with our mistakes that we did in the past, and our faults. Admitting to ourselves and to the Higher Power the nature of our faults will help us to get free of them.

This step also includes admitting in the presence of another person of our mistakes. It is important to choose a person who you can rely on, who is understanding and not judicial in order to complete this step.

It is especially important step if we take into account that an addicted person lives in denial of his real condition and he is generally unwilling to admit that he is addicted. This denial is what keeps the addict going on with his addiction and his selfishness.

This step helps us cope with denial and raise the awareness of defects and shortcomings.

Step 6: In this step we show for the first time a willingness to let the Higher Power take away our character defects. These defects are those character traits that went beyond all normal proportion and became extreme and damaging to us and to everyone around us. It's not enough to know that we have character faults that have led us to bad character traits in the past. We need to be willing to free ourselves from them. There are some of us who are too scared of the unknown to try and get rid of these damaging character traits. In this step we internalize the premise that after we have made an effort to free ourselves from these character faults, we will suffer much less from what we are going through in our current situation. We will not let fear of change weaken our resolve.

With this step we show openness to deep changes with the help of a Higher Power.

We are ready to leave a familiar comfort zone. We understand that in order to change ourselves, our own will is not enough? We need to give our character faults over to a Higher Power with the knowledge that only with help can we make an opportunity to get rid of these faults.

The rule here is not to use force to push these faults of character away from us but to allow the Higher Power to enter our lives more and more. At the same time, step by step we will develop our taking of personal responsibility over ourselves and our actions.

Step 7: In this step we humbly request from the Higher Power to remove these faults that amplified our addiction. We are aware that only with the help of that Higher Power we will be able to reach this goal.

After endless attempts to control our faults with our own will, we understand that only if we let a Higher Power work in our life these faults will be removed. These are the faults that fed our internet addiction and led us to it. In this step we don't stand and wait to find out how our faults will disappear. We choose to let the Higher Power give us wisdom that will lead us on a better path and in this way our faults will no longer control us and our lives. When we request strength from the Higher Power, we do it with feeling of helplessness in front of our addiction.

In a state of active addiction, we lack inner serenity. We find ourselves constantly striving for social affirmation and new stimuli on the internet and we have no peace of mind. In the seventh step, we believe in the Higher Power and the help that this higher Power can give us, and in this way we can achieve more inner serenity. From a ceaseless race of obsessive surfing on the internet, we reach safe shores that can give us a feeling of support and inner quiet.

Step 8: In this step we will try to ask forgiveness from the people we have hurt. It is precisely at this point that we begin to repair the damage that we caused, that we will be able to continue the process in a state of freedom and out of choice. It could be that we have hurt other people in the past. Memories of this can come up in to our consciousness and make us feel guilt and remorse. The 12 Steps are built in a way that leads us on a path of freedom from the past so we can live properly in the present. In order to get free of these feelings, we have to make a list of all the people we hurt in the past. Instead of feeling like victims of other people's acts or victims of circumstance, we start to take responsibility for ourselves and our lives, and all the wrongs in the past. In this step, we will also make the effort to get rid of resentment and anger as these feelings are not good for the freedom of the soul. It is very important for the healing process we are going through each step.

Step 9: In this step, after we prepared a list of the people we hurt (in Step 8), we get ready to say sorry to them. This task can seem especially difficult, but it gives the strongest evidence that we are serious about changing our life. Our thought and behavior patterns in the past perhaps hurt people around us unintentionally. The egocentricity and self absorption blinded us to how much we were hurting others. It could be that we neglected family members while surfing the net obsessively or hurt them in indirect ways.

This step reinforces our sensitivity to others and their needs. A person with self-respect knows how to respect others. By asking forgiveness from people we have hurt, we increase our self-respect as people.

One needs a lot of courage to go and apologize to someone we hurt. Asking for strength from a Higher Power can help us overcome the difficulty of this step.

Our approach to the subject is not depending on the reaction of the people or the result. Our personal responsibility is only to carry out the task and ask for forgiveness. The reaction to this act is not our responsibility.

Step 10: At this stage there are probably signs of change that began with the previous steps. But we cannot always change past patterns within a short time. Sometimes there is falling. The tenth step creates the awareness that this can happen. Immediate awareness of our actions and their consequences is necessary. This awareness is very important so we don't get swept back into our past patterns that can pull us straight back into addiction. We examine our thoughts and day to day behavior and check if it fits our new way of life. In this step we will try to develop a good, efficient sense of self inspection. Even if this does not happen, we will have the power to get right back on track. This ability to admit in mistakes that we made can give us a lot of strength.

Step 11: The contact with a Higher Power is emphasized in the 12 Steps Program. In this step we try to internalize the fact that we are not alone in the world. Our goal is to strive for a conscious, open contact with our Higher Power.

We are no longer alone; by prayer and meditation we constantly improve our link with G-d. In this step we ask through prayer to have the strength for what we need to do. Before we were aware of our Higher Power, we relied only on our own strength. This caused us to fail again and again. In this step we ask for a completely different kind of strength. We ask for strength to act according to the will of G-d. We understand that the will of the Higher Power is good and beneficial for us and we do this from our own free will.

Step 12: The twelfth step is known as a step for preservation. This step helps to conserve all the work we have done in previous steps. Carrying this message to other addicts and giving help to those who want help. We are required to use our special talents, each one in his field in order to help addicts to the internet. Carrying the message that there is a way out of addiction, is very important. It is important to emphasize that the steps need to be done in a group and with experienced person guide. This way you will get the maximum from the steps.

Positive Motivation

In order to win the battle with internet addiction we have to put more happiness and positive thinking into our life. When we are full of happiness we feel free from troubles and worries and thus full of enthusiasm and vitality to do things more efficiently. On the other hand, when we are experiencing emotional discomfort, it will be more difficult to do our daily tasks.

"Okay," you argue, "I understand how important it is to be happy but what can one do if it is hard sometimes?"

There are objective reasons that do not always add to happiness. The debts to the bank, a health problem, marital problems, difficulties at work, all these can definitely over cloud our happiness.

In order to leave the cycle of negative feelings that feed the addiction, we must first decide that we choose to be happy! To be really happy is first of all a matter of choice. Conscious choice has a huge power.

Here you will surely ask: "Who doesn't want to be happy?"

You'd be surprised to hear, but there are people who would prefer to withdraw into negative feelings. They feel that they are life's victims. This feeling leads them to feel that they are not responsible for their lives as they are victims of circumstance.

Happiness helps to motivate us to positive actions. It does not let us sink into a feeling that we are victims. When we are happy we take responsibility for ourselves and our lives. When we live with a conscious choice to be happy, we can accept any event and any difficulty in life and deal with it properly. Happiness fills us with the positive feelings. This way resentment will not control us. Being busy with resentments keeps us locked in the past with all its negative aspects. This in itself steals a lot of our positive energy from us and we have no room in our minds to do what is good and beneficial for us. This can be compared to a swamp that the more we struggle to get out of, the more we sink into it. But happiness lets us look forward, to focus on the future and to anticipate that it will be positive and profitable for us. Thought creates reality. It can be prophesy that fulfills itself. When we are full of happiness, we will focus on the positive and not on the negative. We will look kindly at other people and try to find constructive, positive solutions to different situations. We see that people who are happy are people who are successful. Their happiness gives them new energy that helps them succeed. People who are happy are more open to making friends and starting relationships, and in contrast, sad people will have a harder time building satisfying and constructive relationships. When a happy person stands before a challenge, he looks forward and focuses on solutions to the difficulties he is facing. A person lacking happiness will focus on past events or the problem itself and not on a solution. All we have to do when starting out is to decide to try and be truly happy, and that we will have a positive approach to life. One of the things that ruin happiness is constant dissatisfaction. A feeling that something is missing in our life. This may be something we cannot always put our finger on. This feeling of dissatisfaction can lead us to a constant chase after thrills. If we choose to be happy, we will feel more satisfied.

And since to be happy is something that depends on our own choice, it doesn't matter what events we go through or what our life circumstances are. Even if the situation is not easy, on the contrary, especially now, happiness will give us new strength to overcome the problems we are facing. In other words, happiness does not have to depend on some outside factor or event. It is dependent only on our decision to be happy in any situation and all the time. Awareness of the constant presence of a higher power, of God can make us happier.